EATING SMALL

Table of Contents

Introduction

Fan Your Motivational Flames

It Is Not Your Fault – The 3 T's

However It Is Your Consequence

Decide To Be Fit

Know A Few Things

Go-To Foods – DREAM Foods

Caution! – POUNDS

Finding Honest John

Believing Honest John

Momentum

Range Theory

The Bounce

Making it Fun and Easy

Breaking Through Plateaus

Controlling Your Self Talk

Affirmations

The Illusion That It Comes Naturally

The Psychology of Weight Gain

Prioritizing Calorie Balance

Some Challenges

The Other Diets

Getting Off Track

Moving It

Visualizing

Music Moves Me – The 3 M's

Keeping a Log

Lifestyles of the Obese and Overweight

The Fit Feeling

Fading Memories of Obesity

Jump Starting

Communicate

FITME

Focus on Your Next Meal

EATING SMALL

Steve Daniel Hansberger

Why should it be important to you to be at your correct weight?

Is this statement true? "The most important thing I will do today is to manage my caloric intake."

Many of us would disagree and say that survival, or serving mankind, or something else is more important. Yet, can you do those other things if you have ill health and are laying in a hospital bed due to an ailment relating to a lack of fitness? What about lost years due to dying early? Could you do those other things if you were more fit?

Everything about our lives is enhanced if we are fit, defining fitness for now as "at our correct weight". Of course, true fitness means more than just being at our correct weight. It also includes nutrition and cardiovascular fitness, but for purposes of this discussion, let's limit it to being at our correct weight. Whether you are a paleo, Atkins, vegan, vegetarian, or whatever kind of nutrition person, being at your right weight affects everything about your life. This includes health, agility, movement, appearance, social interaction and our political lives. That is what people are saying about us when we are not around, our image and reputation. All of these things that are affected by being at our correct weight lead to a direct effect on our sex appeal. As a direct result, this all results in a negative impact on our economic effectiveness. So, being at our right weight is a huge factor in our effectiveness at getting what we want out of this short life. It enhances our ability to get what we want, to be effective. Try this acronym out:

"FITME-Fit me Is Truly More Effective".

Here are a few more...

"FREE" – "Fitness Really Enhances Effectiveness"

"FEED" – "Fitness Enhances Effectiveness Dramatically"

Introduction

"Love yourself enough to enjoy your BEST life at your ideal weight."

"If not now, when? When will I make my body fit and thereby enjoy my best, fit bodied life?"

"I make it easier to be effective by maintaining my correct body weight."

Somebody loves you enough to buy this book for you. Possibly it is you that loves you and you acquired it for yourself. Perfect! Either way, I wrote it for you.

I also wrote it for me. Until I learned what follows, I struggled with managing my weight. In the past, even when I lost weight, it was only with great effort to modify what I ate plus lots of exercise and then I went back up again as soon as I stopped the "diet" and/or stopped exercising. So now I have this fitness handbook to refer to should I ever lose my way again.

I also wrote this book for others as I have lost too many friends to obesity and its effects such as diabetes, cancer and heart disease, not to mention the miserable existence of living in an overweight body. I have sensed and heard them discuss their unhappiness, loneliness, desperation, frustration and their problems, many of which were directly related to their bodies being overweight. I wrote this to help all of us to attain and maintain our appropriate weight. As always, **you should check with your physician and follow their direction**.

So with that in mind, may I offer an opinion and some experiences on the attainment of the goal of weight control? This view comes to you from me, from my mind and not from my body. I differentiate between mind and body because it is crucial that your conscious mind take control of your eating and drinking. That means your mind telling your body what to do in spite of your body telling your mind, "I like this so keep eating." Even as I write this sentence, there is ice cream in my fridge that I will eat, but I will not eat it right now because earlier today, I ate enough for this hour of my day which is 12:44pm. My mind is in conscious control of my caloric intake, which is my eating and drinking. You too will have to make conscious decisions to manage your caloric balance.

Now I know this does not sound like rocket science but there is so much more to this, obviously, as 2/3 of Americans live in overweight bodies to their own detriment. What is it that is going on?

Part of it is taste addiction combined with inattention to caloric consumption due to an inadequate prioritization of this part of our lives. So let's fan the flames of motivation so we prioritize calorie balance properly.

Fan Your Motivational Flames

Would you pull up to your workplace with a tanker trailer carrying enough gasoline to power your car for a year? If you did, you would probably be looked at with amazement because everyone knows there is gasoline at the gas station on almost every major intersection and there is absolutely no need to carry that surplus around.

Yet we carry in some cases over a year's worth of food stored under our skins as fat. Now, why do we do this? It's certainly not because there is a food shortage. As we all know, there is a place to eat, just like with gasoline, on almost every major street corner. It is plentiful and it is everywhere. It is not because we are worried about missing tomorrow's meal. We are not preparing for the apocalypse or a reality show. There is something else going on here. What is it?

It is taste addiction combined with inattention. Unlike other harmful addictions like drugs, we have to eat on a daily basis. So this means we have to manage this addiction on a day in, day out basis while we continue to dance with the devil and eat our daily meals. So there is no "cold turkey" quitting. We have to eat and so we have to learn to manage our use of food. Even more difficult, we have to do so in a social environment with other food users. This is sort of like trying to minimize our abuse of an addictive substance while still hanging out with other addicts. A bit tricky to do so! More about managing social eating later.

Another motivator to lower our weight is the people we care about. Have you lost a loved one early to smoking cigarettes which led to emphysema, cancer, etc.? What about drug addiction? Does obesity affect longevity, quality of life, and our relationships with others? Of course it does. Denying your loved ones your companionship by dying young is one of the negatives of obesity. Are there other social, economic and personal consequences to obesity that are not mentionable out of respect for and sensitivity to others?

It Is Not Your Fault – The 3 T's

Have you ever stopped to think about the fact that you are descended from a continuous string of survivors, starting with your parents, grandparents, great-grandparents, and so on? If one of them had not lived long enough to have the next generation's child, you would not be here. A perfect chain of survivors all the way back to the beginning. It is truly amazing. Maybe one or more of them barely made it and only did so as a result of overeating and thereby retained the genes that give us our propensity for overeating. Either way, let's consider what the history of your ancestor's food and drink is.

Starting somewhere around 10,000 years ago, the really big animals such as the wooly mammoth, cave hyena and others died out. If we assume 20 years per generation, that is only 500 generations before you and I. Around that same time, we transitioned to living in bigger groups with agriculture and animal herding and away from being tribal hunter gatherers. These progressively bigger groups enjoyed specialization and agriculture improved. Soon we were growing food in plentiful quantities in the river valleys, for example in the Tigris and Euphrates river area in present day Iraq. Cities grew up and even more specialization occurred.

The spice trade flourished and our food grew ever tastier as a result. Over time, we went from eating meat and gathered fruits and vegetables, to eating production from crops and domesticated animals. Still later, in the last millennium, we discovered potatoes, corn and sugar cane in the new world and brought them to Europe. Did you know as recently as 500 years ago we sweetened with honey and apple juice and did not have sugar? That is only 25 generations ago! In the last hundred years, we have seen our food researched and experimented with to further the goal of making it ever more appealing. So now, our food is plentiful, well prepared and incredibly tasty. Our grocery stores are unbelievably full of variety in produce and all kinds of delicious processed foods. In the last 4 or 5 generations, advertising has been very effective to make it all so desirable.

As our bodies have not changed that much in 500 generations, our food requirements have not changed that much either. However, with the above changes in agriculture and society, our food supply has changed dramatically. More carbohydrates than ever, combined with tastiness at a level we have never seen before. Freshness at its highest level with our restaurants and markets. Temperature, taste and texture at their maximums.

To make things worse, we are bombarded by constant commercials and other advertising pushing more and more food on us. These are extremely well designed to make us say yes to more food. Think of pizza commercials for example as a hard to resist suggestion to our minds. Notice what percent of the ads you see are food or drink related. This advertising not only appeals directly to our hunger but also to our lifestyle, as if buying their product will create a desirable change. It is no wonder we are overeating, in general.

In addition, visual stimuli trigger our eating habits. As we drive down the street, we are bombarded with, for example, the golden arches which trigger in our mind a memory of the taste of whatever our favorite meal is. The

French fries, perhaps, the salt, the texture, the heat, the feeling of them being chewed in our mouths, the salt and potato flavor satisfying our taste buds. Maybe it is the ketchup and mustard of a hamburger mixed with the juices of the meat and the cheese as we bite into the soft warm bun. The combination of those tastes, temperatures and textures in our mouths create a feeling that we desire. It is actually a proven fact that pleasurable eating releases chemicals in our brain that make us happy.

I use fast food only as an example, pick any of your favorites. It may not be fast food for you, it could be home cooking, that you cook yourself. The point is it is our memory of the 3 T's, these tastes, textures and temperatures that make us want them again and again and again.

As a result of the 3 T's we sometimes eat too much at one sitting. Portion sizes and meal sizes in America are enormous compared to European and other countries. If you eat out often and finish your plate or the chips, etc., you are guaranteed to gain weight. You must get a to-go box or waste the remainder. Our weight goes up and our weight gain is due to over indulgence of our addiction to these memories of taste, texture and temperature, combined with the fact that the accumulation of the stored fat is very subtle. It is accumulative but in so many cases, unnoticed. Even as we weigh on the scale it is usually very gradual.

All this goes with a more sedentary lifestyle as we are in "the office" vs hunting and gathering. Consider also the lifestyle of our ancient ancestors. We know there were bears four times the size of grizzly bears, cave hyenas, very large feline predators, not to mention very large ancestors to wolves, hunting in packs. What do you think happened to the overweight humans who moved slowly or with less agility? Personal combat and group combat are much less likely than in our past. Running faster than the other guy (a little joke) is rarely needed for physical survival. These motivators have receded as we have become more civilized and dominant among the various species.

So we are eating more, burning less calories and require less fitness for survival. All that makes it not your fault. However...

It IS Your Consequence

"The cost of overeating is extremely high."

When one does overindulge, storage occurs. We become fat. Our intestines will mindlessly absorb whatever we put into our mouths regardless of the status of our fat surplus. Obesity is to our detriment and ultimately to our early demise. Diabetes, arteriosclerosis, COPD, heart attack, stroke, cancer and other physical ailments are directly associated with obesity. There are other costs to our energy level, movement, appearance, self-esteem, finances and almost every aspect of our lives.

We must take responsibility for exercising conscious control of our caloric intake to immediately shed any surplus weight. To not do so is to end up with an accumulation of stored calories in the form of fat all over our bodies. Obesity, or morbid obesity, indicates that one is not exercising control of their caloric intake and is indulging their desire for excess food and/or drink. That means the 3 T's, taste, texture and temperature. This indicates a lack of self control and therefore has social, political and thereby financial implications, too.

We thicken up and affectionately name our overweight body areas such as our middles, our bellies, rear ends and our handles. We sometimes eat to the point that we are literally so fat that we are clumsy. Have you ever dreaded that you would drop something at work and have to pick it up, knowing how awkward you look getting down to pick it up on one knee because you are obese? Do your knees, hips, back or feet give you pain because you are overweight?

It is all self-imposed. Significantly overstoring calories is not an efficient state of being a human. You will be encumbered by that poundage throughout your day, and it will make you tired more quickly, less flexible, less agile, and less capable of doing more work and may put your safety at risk due to your impaired movement. As an employee, it is a competitive disadvantage to over indulge on your food. Therefore, it can affect you economically as well. It has far reaching implications upon your social life as well as many other things. To not address obesity leads to a less than optimal quality life and early death. That is the simple truth.

What about physical ability to fight? I saw a reality show contestant state flat out that due to her high weight, running was not an option, so she had to be prepared to fight. She was located in the presence of wildlife danger including wild bears. Do we make ourselves a target for predators by being overweight? I bet our hunter gatherer ancestors thought so. Think of the saying, "I don't have to be faster than the bear, I just have to be faster than you!" Think also of the competitive environment that is today's workplace. You worked hard on your education, exercising self-control to study. So bring your best game to the competition. Be fit and, as a result, be more effective at getting what you want.

Decide To Be Fit

"If not now, then when will I make my body fit and thereby enjoy my best, most effective life?"

Do you comb your hair, brush your teeth and bathe regularly? Of course you do! Do you change the oil in your car, keep it maintained with good tires on it? If you like, think for a moment about why you do all of these things.

Maintaining our weight at the proper level is something that is also important. We need to be committed to and diligent about taking conscious decision making control over our caloric intake. Managing our eating/drinking and exercising that control before every meal and especially during the meal.

It is truly a mental focus challenge! As one of my sons told me, "I've had cheese enchiladas, I know what they taste like and I'll have them again, but not right now." He makes a decision about the quantity of calories that he puts in his stomach, per unit of time. He is at or near his correct weight. I've noticed that when I bite into a meal that is particularly tasty that I can literally lose focus on the fact that I am over my weight target and that I need to be reducing weight by eating less than my daily caloric burn rate. I then blow my daily caloric intake number right there, in that one sitting. This occurs just because something is that tasty. It can be pizza, Italian food, dessert, or for me it is typically saucy and/or spicy things. One of my potential weaknesses is ice cream. Do I put two tablespoons in a cup or do I fill the cup and eat it? Do I go back for seconds? Potato chips, spicy but relatively dry, are so flavorful that you can eat 2000 calories just grazing out of the bag while watching TV or surfing the web. One of my most fit female 60 plus year old clients admits to this weakness for chips. Yet she is at her perfect weight. She makes a decision about her caloric intake but knows her weakness.

So how do we get control and not forget to make a conscious decision when faced with our taste addictions? In my case, I had to make it my top priority because anything less was not working.

Know A Few Things

"There is nothing I will do today that is more important than managing my caloric intake."

I repeat the above every morning and all during the day, especially at meal time and during meals. I know other things are important, but you must be alive to do them and obesity is deadly.

Know you are ready for the good fit life.

Know your daily caloric burn rate.

Know your weaknesses and avoid them or at least be cautious with them.

Know calorie counts of your foods.

Know to say this to yourself – "I will enjoy more of this at another time."

Know the 5 bite rule! Remember the next bite will taste the same as the last one. Take 5 bites of the same taste, then pause and reflect on whether to have 5 more bites. This is especially effective with chips. Only 5 before you pause and make a decision, fitness or more of the 3T's.

Think half a fist to 2/3 of a fist as the appropriate volume per meal.

Go To Foods – DREAM Foods

Know your DREAM foods. DREAM stands for Durable, Repeatable, Enjoyable, Available and Measurable. These will be the foundation of your effort to reach and maintain your right weight.

As I approach my correct weight, I look back and realize that 90% of what made this progressively easier and easier over time were my "go to" foods. These are the foods that worked for me. They made hitting my caloric targets at meal time almost effortless. By effortless, I mean not having to exercise a lot of self-discipline. In fact, I look forward to indulging in meal time and am completely satisfied by my meals!

Now I realize that each of us has different "go to" foods. Some of us like one thing, others prefer something else. What should a "go to" food look like? "Go to" foods are what I call DREAM foods. Again, D is for Durable, R is for Repeatable, E is for Enjoyable, A is for Affordable, and M is for Measurable. Let's go into more detail on each of these.

Durable means it stays with you. The problem with sugar and "fast" carbs is that you are hungry again within an hour! Of course, they also spike your blood sugar and, as a result, have harmful effects if you eat or drink more than a small portion of fast carbs. Many of my durable foods are real meats, not eggs or beans or even hamburger. Eggs just are not durable, but I love them and eat them at times. Beans and hamburger are protein rich but turn to mush too quickly in my system and so just don't have the "hang time" I seek in a durable meal.

So for me, durable means unprocessed steak, chicken and seafood. I like it hot in temperature and spicy with garlic salt, cracked black pepper and some jalapeno type heat but you can eat it without these.

Repeatable means I can repeat the meal a thousand times, just like a step of walking can be repeated. It needs to be easy to repeat the food. If I have to make a big effort to prepare or obtain it, forget it. That is not repeatable.

Enjoyable means I love it. It satisfies my need for taste, texture and temperature, the 3 T's. In short, I can't get enough of it. Remember, these foods will be repeated many, many times and thereby make this journey easy. So you have got to love your DREAM foods, your "go to" foods.

Affordable means I can afford it on a daily basis if I desire it that often.

Measurable is the biggie! Know how many calories are in it. There has to be an easy portion control to really make it easy. This means the opposite of a buffet, which is big trays of unknowable volume of your favorites. Measurable means portioned! So for example, a 1 pound T-bone steak is measurable, 16 ounces times 40 calories equals 640 calories, less the bone. This is not a bad calorie count for such a large durable meal. I save half for later or share it. Another modular food is a drumstick or a chicken thigh. So is a piece of shrimp or a filet of fish.

One of my favorite DREAM foods has been beef and chicken tacos with no high calorie add-ons. That means no for beans or guacamole, but yes for low calorie vegetables added, like peppers. Indulge yourself occasionally in the no items. I found over time that if I eat one taco per meal, which is about 300 calories, I lose weight. If I eat two, or 600 calories, I maintain my weight. Three or more, or 900+ calories, and I gain weight. Simple, easy. No big effort except the effort required to eat only one. Over time, this DREAM food made this super easy and it got easier as the weeks passed. It became a habit to eat small. Durable, Repeatable, Enjoyable,

Available and Measurable. DREAM foods! Know yours.

Caution! POUNDS

Over time, I have learned to avoid, except occasionally, what I call POUNDS. The following situations are what I mean by POUNDS. Can you tell I love acronyms? They make it easy for me to remember things.

P is for Processed. Even a hamburger patty is processed. 80/20 or 90/10, it is still already shredded. Why is that bad? It pretty much dissolves in your mouth. This means no "hang time", no "durability", or at least not as much as non-processed meat. Other processed foods include pizzas, most fast foods, pastas, breads, etc. If you read the labels and it has a bunch of words in it that you don't recognize, it is probably processed. These chemicals may have side effects as my mom said they always do. So I lean toward fresh vegetables, which I think of as unprocessed herbs and spices. Think about the fact that most of your herbs and spices are ground up plants. So diversify your herbs and spices with some that are not processed! Yes, I mean veggies. Think of green beans as a spice that just hasn't caught on for whatever reason. An entire can of green beans is 70 calories and is quite a lot of food. It makes a great quick snack, especially if you throw a little meat in. It is good cold, too. On the meat front, sausage is processed and is 90 calories per ounce vs 20 for shrimp and 40 for beef! So if you eat the same amount you are eating vastly more calories with sausage. Processed also can mean fillers like gluten and fast carbs.

The O in POUNDS means overly tasty. If something is overly tasty it could spell POUNDS on you! Watch out. Especially in social eating out settings as the restaurants really make it tasty, don't they? Of course! They want you to return.

U means unpicked, meaning "I did not pick this restaurant, appetizer, entrée, thing in the refrigerator, etc." This one is big. How many times have you been out to eat and they put chips and salsa in front of you? Or somebody orders queso for the table, or nachos, or guacamole? Or you look in the fridge and you find your favorite ice cream that you did not buy? You get the picture. If you did not pick it, it could become POUNDS on you! Perhaps you should have them take it away immediately, move it away from you and/or speak up kindly. Develop the ability to cope with this situation. Handle it. Be effective.

N means not durable. Think of a donut and how it doesn't stick to your ribs as compared to some chicken which does. If it is not durable and leaves you hungry again in an hour, it could put POUNDS on you.

D is the most important letter in POUNDS and it stands for distracted. There is nothing that puts more POUNDS on us than eating while we are distracted. This means eating while we are doing something else. Social eating, eating while watching TV, reading, driving, playing, working or performing any activity that distracts us can put POUNDS on you. I think for me it started with reading the back of the cereal box while I ate cereal in the morning as a kid. Remember to stay focused and make good decisions about your caloric intake.

S is for social eating. Social eating has been my biggest challenge as it is the most frequent cause when I over eat. Partially it is because I am distracted while I am eating socially as I love to visit. It frequently entails all of the POUNDS elements, Processed, Overly tasty, Unpicked (think appetizers and chips), Not durable and Distracted. In short, social eating is probably our biggest challenge. May I also add sauces, spicy, syrups, salt and sweets to the "S" list? We can call them the 5 S's. Any of these can spell trouble. So exercise caution and be prepared to be strong in your decisions when you are presented with POUNDS situations! Label foods that you have in your home if you have to - "POUNDS!" - to remind you to be cautious with them.

Finding Honest John

For me, it came like an avalanche. One day I woke up and could not believe what I had allowed my body to become. It was similar to that dream I frequently have of suffocating, restricted, unable to move, barely able to catch a breath. In retrospect, I think I was close to dying. I could not stop it, it seemed. One day, I got lucky and found a friend who would not lie to me. That friend was a triple beam balance scale that weighed to my full weight and it said the same thing to me every time I stepped on it. It told me what I actually weighed. No leaning to vary the reading. It gave me my accurate weight every time. I called it "Honest John". Finding Honest John was the beginning of success. It is crucial to find your own Honest John and to weigh yourself at the same time, in the same clothes, every day. For me, that is upon waking after dawn, usually around 6:30 am in my sleepwear.

Believing Honest John

Over time, I learned that Honest John was providing me with the truth about my actual weight and I came to believe it. I learned that if I stepped on Honest John the next day and I was heavier, I had eaten too much over the previous 24 hours. If I stayed the same, I was at a balance, maintaining my previous day's weight. If I lost weight, I had eaten less than I had burned, calorically. Now of course this is not perfectly accurate on a daily basis as there are factors like hydration and food in process, but generally, this was the truth. I realized all I had to do was find an HONEST accurate scale, weigh every day at the same time in the same clothes, and believe what it said. That is, up equals too much, down is too little and no change equals caloric balance. The next thing to do is to figure out a way to start shedding pounds.

Momentum

Once you obtain and decide to believe Honest John, and you weigh every day, same time, same clothes, you may find that you are not losing weight and that you may still be gaining!

Eat smaller. As you eat progressively smaller until the weight gain stops you will feel in control of your weight, perhaps for the first time. No tricks, no fad diets, no skipping the carbs, just controlling your caloric balance on a daily and even per meal basis. Eating small. You will then say to yourself, if I can stop the gaining, I can reduce my intake further and actually reduce my weight. That's what I did.

You will start knowing the calories in everything you eat and drink and know your count as the day progresses. That's right, breakfast was 300, lunch was 400, so I'm at 700 going into late afternoon, as an example. As a result, you will come to know your daily caloric burn rate, which is how many calories you can have without gaining or losing weight. For me, this started out as close to 2750 and as I lost that first 50 pounds, it went down to more like 2250. It will change with weight loss as you need fewer calories to carry less weight. However, your energy level will improve so your activity will increase and this leads to more calories burned.

Next, divide your daily caloric burn rate into your meals, snacks, late night indulgences, per day. Be realistic in your planning! You cannot eat all of your calories before 10am and expect to not eat for the rest of the day. It is just not likely to happen with our social eating and so forth. I usually skip breakfast, eat about 400 to 600 calories for lunch, about the same for dinner and then have a small bowl of cereal or something to add some fiber to move my system. I am rarely hungry at lunch time even though I skip breakfast and have not eaten in 15 hours.

My goal is to lose approximately 1/3 of a pound per day. Since there are approximately 3500 calories in a pound of fat that means about 1166 calories below my daily burn rate, each day. Since my daily burn rate is about 2250, that's about 1100 calories per day. Why do I target that amount of weight loss? I have found that is the most I can do on a sustained basis. Any more weight loss per day and I am inconsistent. In fact, even at that rate, I still have what I call eating days, when I exceed my burn rate, sometimes by a thousand calories or more. I have learned not to overreact or give up or get negative, I just resume eating small.

Sometimes, I'll skip the next meal, usually breakfast, as for me the excess usually happens in a social setting at dinner time. After all, I am not a machine!

When I do overeat as defined by exceeding my daily caloric burn rate, and do so frequently enough to not move Honest John downward, I am creating what I call a plateau or a bounce. I get to a level and can't seem to get below it. I bounce and I dip and I bounce and I dip. It does happen! What's going on is complacency. I get comfortable. I have to resume fanning the flames of motivation, usually with new goals and visualizations, new targets. I need a new "range"! Again, the question is **"If not now, when will I make my body fit and thereby enjoy my best, fit bodied life?"** Fan those flames of motivation. See yourself at the lower weight. Visualize yourself enjoying your best life at a fit weight.

Range Theory

What I call range theory is the idea that people who control their weight have a range in which their weight moves. Now for many of the obese people, they do not have a range and more or less eat what they want, when they want and as much as they want. However, most folks who have some type of management of their weight operate in a certain range. This means that when they get to the high end of their weight range they take action to address it, whether that is to eat small, stop eating, cut out the carbs, exercise more, or any one of various approaches to move their weight downward. Once they hit the bottom of their range, their motivation weakens and they become more complacent about their weight and they tend to cycle in that range.

Range should be limited to a max of about 10 pounds. This includes bounces, salt, food in process, dehydration, over and undereating.

How do we move our range as our weight moves downward? How do we refocus ourselves to push it progressively lower all the way to fitness? Likewise, how do we manage to not become anorexic or bulimic and go past the point of fitness to being too thin?

The Bounce

Let's examine the "bounce" which occurs at the bottom of our "range" and the cause of the bounce which is complacency. It is basically an overeating day.

This is how it happens. You are losing weight, doing well. One day as you are getting complacent and you overindulge, possibly due to a social outing or just letting go. What happens then is you don't truly gain a lot that day, but because the way your body works, holding water and all, you will see a gain of a pound or two the next day.

In my experience, when I "bounce", meaning go up 3 pounds from an eating day, I know I did not really gain 3 pounds which is 10,500 calories. My excess eating is usually about 1000 calories over my burn rate. However, even after I allow a day or two to rebalance, I find that my weight loss momentum has taken a hit. It takes a few days of staying with eating small to resume the decline. So the price of indulgence is usually about a 5 or 6 day period with no loss of weight. This is a hit to the mental side and so I think it is worth it to avoid it as much as I can.

Complacency is what we are fighting as we try to get all the way down to our correct body weight range. So stay motivated! One piece of advice is to try not to eat so little that you become hungry. Don't try to do too much too fast. One third of a pound per day is my personal maximum that works on an ongoing basis, and I still overeat at times.

Making it Fun and Easy

To add some fun to it, why not think of what you eat and what you expend in exercise in terms of calories? So instead of saying "I had French fries for lunch." Say, "I had 300 calories of French fries for lunch." Likewise, instead of saying "I walked 3 miles today". Say, "I walked 15000 feet, which is approximately 6000 steps, or 600 calories, which is my estimate for my body." This puts it in its true calorie balance format and makes it easier to monitor your caloric balance, per day and per meal. So if you go over, you simply plan to go for a walk to compensate! Fun and easy.

Here is another way to make it fun and easy. Eat what you like, just limit the quantity. I had a half a taco today for breakfast and it was more than adequate with the sauce, the texture and temperature. It was so delicious and I really did not have a desire to have more as it was satisfying. I am thinking that for many of us, overeating has a lot to do with the desire to fill that desire for whatever it is that makes us unsatisfied. If you are eating something that you really like and that your body is desiring, I'm going to go out on a limb a little bit and say maybe that is what you should be eating. This taco satisfied my body's desire for fats, spice, meat and carbs with the tortilla. I dunked it all in a quite spicy and enjoyable green sauce. The point is satisfaction of the taste appetite is not a function of quantity, it's more a function of satisfying what it is that you want. Just eat small.

Again, I think that it is important to be mindful to not overindulge on those foods that are our weaknesses, that which we think is delicious. Like saucy foods, which make all of our mouths water, we have to know our weaknesses as we try to eat small. Even now I can think of some foods that make me salivate. Try to be particularly mindful of portion control with foods that you know to be your weaknesses.

Breaking Through Plateaus

As I examined a plateau of 6 months duration that I experienced, I realized it was due to complacency. The things which motivated me at 40 pounds heavier were no longer motivators! I had to find new motivators, such as losing inches on my waist, not so much about health as about appearance. I needed to transition from losing weight from an obese body to losing weight from an overweight body. Perhaps a new motivator would be having my pants or one's dress size going down for some new clothes. Perhaps the motivators would be looking better, moving better, having more energy, being physically more attractive not only to others but to myself. Another would be feeling that I look good both in clothes and undressed. Find your motivator and be prepared to come up with new ones as you lose weight!

So just like at the beginning, I decided to try eating smaller, to modify my eating volume from my plateau level to less. I went from 3 tacos at lunch to 2 and then to 1 taco. The result was a weight loss of 7 pounds within 2 or 3 weeks. I broke through the plateau and it felt great! It happened one meal at a time, just by focusing again on the basic premise of this book, Eating Small, which is to "eat small."

But was it just as easy as that? How did I summon the will power to eat less, again? After all, the plateau had been caused by complacency, showing itself as eating 3 tacos for lunch instead of 2 for maintenance or 1 for weight loss, as I said earlier in the book! I knew it when I ate the 2nd and 3rd tacos that this would mean a lack of weight loss that day. So why was I doing the additional eating? Well as you know it was because I enjoy the taste, texture and temperature of the tacos! I had stopped eating small and was eating medium and large, resulting in a maintenance of my weight, not reduction. I was indulging myself because I was complacent about my weight. I needed to do something to break through that plateau, to regain my motivation to take it down further. I needed to change my self-talk.

Controlling Self Talk

I simply made a decision to eat small again on my next meal. I was in fact tired of the plateau, the lack of movement as I still weighed too much! There was no question that I wanted to lose more. In addition, I had watched others that I know lose 50 pounds on other low carb diets and then bounce back up by 20 pounds or more. I knew I was on the right track with this eating small thing because I had reached a plateau, not bounced back up. So I knew that all I had to do was to eat small again, meal by meal, and my weight would go on down. There was no need to make a big deal out of it. Just eat small my next meal.

Many of us have not been taught how to manage our caloric intake, so we have to learn to do it on our own or somewhere else. On the contrary, do you remember, "Finish your plate! There are kids starving in the world!" Many of us have had verbal and sometimes hurtful quips thrown at us from family, friends and others, such as "that last 5 pounds looks really good on you" as one of my former male employers said to me one day. As with all criticism that attacks the person and not the behavior, this type of experience can be damaging to our self image and thereby have the opposite effect, and get us wrapped around the axle with our internal dialogue. Try to not let that happen and make your self talk affirmative and positive, such as "I enjoy an empty stomach. I can move better. I can breathe better." Take a to-go box or leave the excess food. You deserve a great life so do it for you! Don't let another person's hurtful comment become your internal self-talk. Take control and select your own positive self-talk.

Affirmations

Affirmations are self-talk statements to yourself that help to create successful attainment. Frequently they take the form of already having achieved the desired outcome even before it is attained. This is also called visualization. Here are some examples:

"I remind myself of the 5 bite rule." That is, 5 bites then pause and reflect on whether to have 5 more.

"I enjoy steadily marching my weight downwards."

"I enjoy mastery of my eating."

"I enjoy losing 1/3 to ½ pound per day, and I realize it is the most I can lose on a sustained basis."

"Nothing tastes as good as being fit feels."

"I enjoy fitting comfortably in my clothes."

"I choose the quality of life that goes with fitness."

"I eat to energize my body."

"I know my caloric burn rate per day."

"I know it's a taste, texture and temperature thing, and I know my weakness foods that provide me with the 3 T's."

"I eat what I want, but I decide in advance how much I will eat and when I will eat it."

"I plan my next meal when I am not hungry.

"I deserve my best life."

"I visualize a quality life for myself."

"I enjoy a pretty much empty stomach." More than anything else in my journey, I have found this to be the key. Eat small. Enjoy whatever you like, but after you eat half a fist of volume, stop. You can and will have more at a different time.

"They are not going to stop making it." For example, ice cream cones, candy, chips, cookies, snacks, etc. Remember it is about balancing intake with your burn rate, so eat small for now and enjoy empty, knowing you will have more later.

"I just go past (ignore) my impulse to eat at times and wait for the next time to indulge." For me, this frequently buys me another 2 to 3 hours between eating. Another way to say this is, "No, for now."

"Drive on by. Right now I am on a roll to get fit." I use this one to avoid my favorite fast foods and those aisles in the grocery store that contain my weakness foods.

"Nothing tastes as good as being fit feels." Did I already say that?

Create your own affirmations that address the unique psychology of your eating.

The Illusion That It Comes Naturally

Do you edit your conversation at meal time? Of course you do! You don't use inappropriate language or crude remarks, monopolize the conversation or act in any way that might offend others, right? You even use table manners! These are all examples of self-control. Recognizing that our eating and drinking require the same self-control and have to be consciously managed is paramount to managing your weight. Our brain does not automatically do the job of managing our caloric intake, unlike our involuntary muscles like our heart beating and lungs breathing which automatically provide the right amount of oxygen to maintain our blood oxygen level. Our bodies DO try to manage our blood sugar levels. However our intestines WILL absorb what we put in them without the intestines making any decision regarding our current calorie storage status. We are fully capable of flooding our blood with sugar simply by overeating, especially fast carbs. However, the body does not send a signal to us that we are storing fat. We tend to look at our food intake with inadequate care and assume that we just eat when we are hungry, 3 meals a day, and that everything is going to be fine. Well, it is not fine. In fact, it can be catastrophic.

We tend to overeat, to over taste, to overindulge and to eat even when we are not hungry, just on impulse and taste addiction. You should also know the difference between being thirsty and being hungry. The whole 3 meals a day thing is arguably a recent development in mankind's history, and was almost certainly not normal in our ancestral millennia, especially before the dawn of agriculture to sustain the ancient cities, to feed the growing populations as hunting was inadequate to feed the masses. We got very, very good at making food tasty. Sauces, spices, temperature, textures and variety as we had never experienced it. So we overindulge our taste buds at the expense of our health and much else.

The Psychology of Weight Gain

If you have allowed yourself to eat too much and thereby to store fat, the overeating is the physical reason why you are overweight. Now there are a lot of mental reasons why that happens. One of them is inattention as described above. It could also be a form of self-destruction, a way to avoid unwanted advances from others, or a response to stress, and many other things.

There are social factors as well! Other people can affect your eating. We tend to become like those we associate with and so we can gain weight as a result of dining with other folks that have poor eating habits. After all, do you always get to pick the restaurant? Their choices affect our choices for where we eat and also what we eat if we are eating at the same table. Think of Unpicked.

Other people can also, if I may use the word, sabotage our weight management. I have watched a TV show in which other people brought pizzas to a person whose weight was over 600 pounds! Talk about enabling! What about the person who buys your favorite POUNDS foods for you and they just show up in your refrigerator? Time to have a little talk with them, right? Again, think Unpicked.

You must honestly and wisely identify and examine each of these issues, one by one, and successfully identify strategies for each. Make a decision on the strategy you will use for each.

The log will help you to more clearly identify these situations and the following will help you to prioritize your caloric management so that you successfully cope with them. The log will also help you to understand the individual psychology of your personal eating. Just use your phone's recorder, quick and easy, any time you have a thought about logging. It is a gift to yourself so do it.

Prioritizing Calorie Balance

"There is nothing I will do today that is more important than managing my caloric balance."

This is my most frequently used affirmation. I repeat this every morning and before meals. I had to do so to keep traction on my weight management journey. I frequently caught myself forgetting to say this when I bounced. Just like with the eating, I didn't make a big deal out of it, I just started saying it again and planned my next meal.

We already make food a very high priority, if we are overweight. I think the current term is "foodie". So plan your next food intake right now. Go with your impulse, whatever you are craving. For me, right this second, it's a sausage, jalapeno and cheese kolache. So here is my plan.

I already ate 900 calories this morning at about 10:30am. By the way, that is too much for this time of day. It was breakfast tacos that I made at home, one of my favs consisting of 4 strips of bacon (50 Cal ea.), 3 scrambled eggs (80 Cal ea.), pico de gallo (negligible Cal) and flour tortillas (2 x 100 Cal each) with approx. 5 cashews and maybe 5 potato chips.

My personal expectation is to lose some weight every single morning weigh in, even if it is just .2 pounds. My daily caloric intake that makes my expectation a reality is about 1500 Cal per day. If I keep it below 1500, I will lose some weight almost every single day, water and food retention being the exception occasionally. I deny myself nothing. I eat exactly what I want to eat. However, I limit the quantity! Try it! It will work for you, too. You will be happy and content with your eating.

Now, these kolaches are to die for, and contain a large sausage, cheese and jalapeno, on homemade bread. I estimate the calories at around 500 for 1 kolache. Late editing note, I don't eat these any more. They are a POUNDS food for me.

Help me here, if I want to see the result tomorrow morning on the scale, how many kolaches can I have? You are exactly correct, one! That's it. Pretty much nothing else today. After I eat it, I will plan a meal for tomorrow. To be honest, I don't eat like this anymore as I prefer to eat smaller meals twice rather than 500 calories in one meal.

So you can see, this is a rate thing! Calories per day. I had lost, at this point, 40 pounds so far doing this. So I did the math, that's 40 pounds x 3200 calories per pound equals 128,000 calories. That's what I had lost. If a whole pepperoni pizza, thin crust, is 2000 calories, then that equals 64 pizzas. So I have eaten 64 pizzas less than what I needed. Or about 85 double meat hamburgers with cheese (1500 each approx.). So you see, overeating really makes a difference quickly, right? You will find that late night eating is worse than morning and midday, so if I'm going to eat some sugar or high carb food, I try to eat it by 2pm and try to be active afterward to burn it off. I make dinner more about protein and slow vegetables, sometimes adding two tablespoons of ice cream or a half cup of cereal with milk. I frequently skip breakfast and occasionally skip other meals. I'm just not feeling the desire to eat when I do so, so it is not a discipline thing. Sometimes I'm just full from the previous meal.

It's not about denying yourself what you want. Resist that impulse to eat and when you think of it again, eat whatever you want, but just stay under your daily caloric burn rate that gets your objective accomplished. Eat small and plan your next meal before you get hungry. Again, I am rarely hungry nor do I crave or deny myself anything that I want to eat.

It's a knowledge thing, too! You must know your daily caloric burn rate and the approximate calories of everything you eat, drink or exercise/work. Know the cost of obesity and make a choice, a decision to be at your right weight.

Some Challenges

Buffets

Ever noticed all the big boys and girls at the "all you can eat" buffets? I was somewhat surprised when I went on a cruise at my own weight management behavior with the all you can eat buffet. Everything I enjoy eating was right there in unlimited quantity. I ate three full breakfasts the first day! It took me a couple of days to re-make the decision to be fit and then restate my mantra and to get back on track. I had just reached a new low when I got on the boat and kind of did a hard push to get there just before boarding, so that helped to trigger my overeating. Slow and steady is better.

The problem with all you can eat buffets is that the portions are not measurable. What I mean is that there are no concise 100 calorie units or any defined caloric portion. Bottom lining it, it is one of the most difficult situations in which to manage my caloric intake. That's the "M" in DREAM, by the way. I was able to lose the four pounds I gained on the cruise within a couple of weeks.

Social Eating

I remember that we never ate out when I was living with my parents. I was overjoyed to discover business lunches. Oh my God! Just like that I went from 28-30" waist to 32".

Social eating throws a few curve balls at us. For one, we are not focused on calorie balance during the meal. Where I live they over portion us like it's our last meal. You MUST request a to go box with every meal out as portions are double or triple your balanced caloric needs.

Another problem is restaurant selection. We don't usually get to pick the restaurant and so frequently we are in a place that is full of our danger foods, those that we are weak for. I'm thinking of chips and salsa or chips and queso in a Mexican food place. I'm full before they bring the entrée! You'll remember that's the "U" in POUNDS. Unpicked.

Eating Fast Food While Driving

Now this is challenging because you are in your favorite restaurant when you order and it is so tempting to add extras to your decision on impulse, as you order. Fast food is loaded with carbs and in general has a short hang time or durability. If I have to do it, I go with a chicken sandwich, no mayo, and I eat the meat only, no bun and no fries. That way, I'm in the 200 calorie range but still tasty. It's okay to do other places if you still hit your calorie balance target for the day. That's the "D" in POUNDS, distracted.

Remember to visually check the breading on the chicken sandwich if you don't go with grilled. Most places cake the breading on and it is full of fast carbs, is very tasty and is processed. That is the P and the O in POUNDS. Watch out! I go with very, very light breading on a real chicken breast.

Aisles in the Grocery Store

There are some grocery store aisles that I frequently avoid because I know my weaknesses are on those aisles. Candy, chips, breads, pastries, ice creams, etc. are examples. You know your own weaknesses. My experience is if I have it in the house, somebody is going to eat it. Guess who that will end up being! Me! If you are tempted to go for it anyway, be careful to put a small portion in a bowl, put the big package back in the pantry or fridge and limit yourself. For me, that's 5 potato chips and I count them. It is two tablespoons of ice cream, medium tablespoons not the gigantic heaping tablespoons. After all, I am fitness bound!

HALT

I have heard that drug treatment programs say don't get too Hungry, Angry, Lonely or Tired, as they perceive those 4 to be triggers for relapsing. It makes sense in a way to use the same guideline for our caloric balance effort. I have found that there are periods of time when I am not at my best, somewhat off track or flat mentally. A lot of times it is due to being one of those four, too hungry, too lonely, but especially tired. I find that my body tends to want to eat when I am very tired. So I make every effort to enjoy my rest instead of overeating. There is also the new term for when we are feeling both hungry and angry. We are hangry.

I have to add thirsty. Don't eat to satisfy thirst, drink instead. Try not to drink your calories. Some obese folks that I know personally still drink sugared beverages all day long. It is hard to lose weight when you are drinking 750 calories per day.

Saboteurs

Perhaps you have some other folks in your life who unknowingly sabotage your calorie balance efforts. Maybe you have a spouse or significant other who always says, "Oh, I'll just have a bite of yours...", as a result, you over order and as you are compelled to clean your plate, because the kids are starving somewhere, you consume more calories than your calorie balance plan was calling for. While they maintain their portion control by nibbling. Others insist on restaurants that just destroy our efforts. I have no answer on that one, as I just endure and then resume my plan. I go a little off plan then just get back on it. I want to socialize, too!

The Big Meal

It all comes down to learning to eat small meals of about 1/3 your daily caloric target. For me, as I am trying to lose 1/3 pound per day, that is about 400 calories per meal. Volume wise, it comes to ½ a fist to 2/3 of a fist of volume. Over time, you will develop this habit, while eating whatever you wish to.

If you blow a meal or a day, who cares? Just get back on it and resume your effort to balance your calories and to enjoy empty. There are few of us that will never have an occasional big meal. After I overindulge, sometimes I will fast for 18 hours or more just to give my system a rest. By fast, I mean from evening until the next day's lunch time. I am truly not hungry at the next meal time, anyway.

I think it is important to note that skipping meals and feeling physically hungry can result in overeating. I rarely am hungry. I also find that overdoing exercise tends to makes me overeat. Better is a couple miles of walking, or just going shopping!

The Other Diets

Everyone has a plan they are on and everyone believes that their plan is the best. However, caloric balance is a never ending self-management effort. It does not end. We must always manage our caloric intake. Our lifelong eating is not a diet, meaning a limited period of time. If I "diet" traditionally, once I go back off of that diet I still have to learn what I am suggesting in this book. That is, to consciously manage my eating and drinking.

I am more likely to keep the weight off permanently if I am eating what I want. That way I learn to exercise control of how much of it I consume. Thereby improving my eating habits so I live and eat the same way after I lose the weight in order to maintain a fit body always.

Please re-read that last paragraph as it is key.

Either way, one has to learn what I am suggesting at the end of the so called diet anyway! Why? Again it is because once they go off the "diet", they will be back to eating what they want! They still have to learn to manage their caloric intake! Usually, they bounce back up as you can't live forever without carbs, or whatever the "diet" omits.

I have proven this as I have kept my weight off while folks on other diets have yes, reduced their weight but they are already bouncing back up. There is no shortcut. Learn and make it your habit to eat small.

So rather than changing your foods temporarily during a "diet" and then trying to transition back to your normal foods and teaching yourself how to maintain your weight while enjoying your normal food preferences, why not simply change the quantity of what you eat, enjoying everything you like now, just eating smaller and make it a lifelong change? Make it the way you live always. That's why eating small works and that's why I wrote this book. It works. Eureka!

Getting Off Track

There will be times when it feels like you blew it and ate too much. It's okay! Just plan your next meal and resume your enjoyment of eating small and slowly drop the pounds you think you gained. The truth is, it takes over 3000 calories to equal a pound so you'd have to really eat large to make even a one pound gain in true weight. Allow for your body to move it all through in a couple of days as you see your weight on the scale. Relax and eat small, each meal.

Moving It

It's an exercise thing too, so move your body. Slow and long is better than intense and short. Intense makes me tend to be voraciously hungry. Slow keeps me more relaxed and balanced in my food decisions. I find mowing the lawn to be a good activity for slow and long. A nice one, two or three mile walk is good for everything, including burning calories, moving the food inside you, endorphin generation, cardio health, muscle and skeletal strength and thinking, too. Unlike running, walking does not bounce your tissues and skin which can cause saggy skin once you lose the weight. I do it pretty much every day. "I enjoy long and short walks." My body burns approximately 1 calorie for every 10 steps, so 5000 steps is 500 calories. 10,000 steps is 1000 calories. You get the point.

Get up off the couch. Move it. Move it. Move it. Dance in your living room! Every little bit helps. "I enjoy moving my body." Wait on yourself instead of asking someone to bring you something. Move.

"Stretching feels good and burns calories."

Let's do a deeper dive on that other aspect to exercise and that is bouncing your tissues. How can it be good for your skin appearance for you to bounce physically as you do in running, while you have a lot of extra fat between your skin and your muscles? Yes, if you run while obese, you are going to stretch that skin with every bounce. Remember, at some point you are going to be slender. Do you want your skin to be stretched out or elastic and tight around you as you become fit? I think a non-bounce exercise is important to this until you get close to your correct weight. So walk, don't run! If you want more cardio, incline walking will give you all you want! I find 115 to 128 pulse rate is plenty. Ease into it, as you don't want to hurt yourself. Listen to your body. Be very gradual and patient as you begin to exercise and follow your doctor's direction before you begin.

Visualization

"The single most important key to achievement is visualization, so visualize yourself already fit."

Visualize yourself at your right weight. I have found visualization to be the most important key to achieving anything. Say it, "I am fit."

Visualization creates a mental picture that your mind will try to turn into reality. So be positive in your thoughts. See yourself enjoying the attainment of your objective in your mind and it will happen. Do not negatively self-talk. If you made a mistake consider it to be developmental. I like to think of everything as developmental and it is! That's why persistence is so important. We are perfecting our effort as we persist.

The 3 M's – Music Moves Me

Use music to empower yourself by playing music that does so. For me, that is anything that makes me feel victorious, energetic and capable. Dancing burns calories!

Keeping A Log

It will help you to keep a log of what you eat, how you are doing, how you feel, DREAM foods and POUNDS situations. You don't have to be obsessive about the log, just be honest with yourself in your notes about what's going on with your thinking and actions. When you review it later you will see patterns that you won't see if you don't keep a log. I am frequently surprised by my notes from over a year ago. I can't believe that I was saying the same things then as I'm saying now, or indulging in things I no longer indulge in. It is amazing how much we do not keep in the front of our mind as you know from looking at old pictures and remembering more details upon doing so. Triggers such as photos and logs enable us to remember the specific details much more effectively.

That's it! Persist! Persist! Persist! By doing it this way you are changing your eating habits in a way that will last your entire life. Eat small and give yourself the gift of a great life at your right weight. Remember:

"If not now, when? When will I make my body fit and thereby enjoy my best, fit bodied life?"

Some of my log follows. If it seems a bit clunky it is because it is my actual log. Notice I still hide my actual weight numbers. Laughing out loud here. For easy quick use, I use my voice recorder on my phone and then transcribe the recording to a word file.

(date)

Weight loss. It is now (date). In the last 10 days to 2 weeks I've had a breakthrough in how to lose weight. Basically, I have to eat a lot less. Not a fist size but half that. Like 2 bacon and 2 eggs for breakfast. Doesn't matter what you eat. Pork rinds seem to have no effect even if you have a half a bag. A quarter of a waffle. Just don't eat too much and the weight will just fall off.

(date)

Today I hit a new record low of (weight). Very satisfied. Same strategy all 3 meals. Eat small. Again pork skins did not seem to hurt. I also had

6 small butterfingers and still lost weight both days. It continues to be about less quantity. For example yesterday I downsized to 1 piece of bacon in my breakfast tacos. For lunch maybe half a hamburger, or split one with someone else. I ate my fries and my partner's fries. Hamburger size was normal. For dinner, I can't remember. But anyway it is working.

(date)

Yesterday went pretty good. I had a large dinner yesterday so I'm up a pound. 2 tacos for breakfast. 2 thin ribeye steaks for lunch. Dinner was 2 hamburger patties with no bun and cheesy pico sauce on top. (weight) this morning.

(date)

(weight). A new low. Consistently moderate meals. I can get into my smaller pants now. Feels a lot better and a lot healthier. As I'm now down 20 pounds, I do not even want to overeat as I feel much better. Why would I want to be back at (weight)? It would take me another 2 or 3 days to get back to (weight). If I just eat moderately, I will go on down. Feel better, sharper and enjoying all the other benefits of being at a lighter weight.

(date)

Another day and my weight is down. I've got a grip on my eating again. I've had a lot of social eating over the last 2 months and I have been at a plateau in my weight loss during that time. Yesterday, I had a spicy chicken patty at 10:30am. At 12:30 I wanted to eat again but was not hungry and took a pass. At 2:30pm I had another spicy chicken patty and that satisfied me. In the evening I ate at about 9pm and made some leftover meat and veggies, 5 strips of bacon, 2 eggs and a bowl of cereal, slightly over a cup with full milk. On the exercise front I walked a lot, probably 4 – 5 miles. The net effect was a 2 pound drop and it feels good. Noteworthy is that I have kept the weight off, even though I have done a lot of social eating. I have done a good job managing my caloric intake. This diet differs from other diets where you starve yourself of something and you end up bouncing as a result.

Keeping a log will improve your ability to manage your caloric intake.

Lifestyles of the Obese and Overweight

The price of obesity is extremely high. If you are 100 pounds overweight, first of all, you are almost certain to die young. **How many obese 80 year olds do you see?** Yes there are a bunch of 50 and 60 year olds that are obese, but it is in those years after 50 that the big killer diseases strike the obese with deadly force. Yes, I'm talking about diabetes, heart disease, strokes, cancer and others, all aggravated by being overweight.

Second, you are going to have major health issues. I have many childhood friends who have popped 100 pounds on seemingly overnight. Next thing I know they are having surgery to remove toes or replace joints or this, that or the other, while they are packing enough surplus energy in the fat cells to nourish them for a year or more without eating. It's sad and totally controllable. The same person at their right weight is likely fine!

As it is crucial, for emphasis I ask you again, **"How many obese 80 year olds do you see out there?"**

Have you ever heard someone say, "He died because he is a food addict." No. They say, "He died of diabetes. Kidney failure. Cancer." They don't say that those were caused directly or indirectly by obesity and food addiction.

However if you die of a drug overdose, they don't say you died of heart failure due to your heart beating too fast or heart attack due to cocaine or crack. They don't say heart attack. They say drugs. So we pin it really aggressively on things like drugs but with food addiction we blame the result instead of the cause.

We talk around it with words like a little chubby, more to love. When you see a person that you consider to be attractive on the street, are they at their correct weight? Are you attracted to the fit, agile, energetic, vigorous and enthusiastic? Is it just their athletic body that is appealing, or is it also the way they move, communicate and their confidence? I discussed this briefly with an overweight friend and she said when you are overweight, people treat you differently. One of my friends who works in HR at a major company had a friend ask her if she would get a better job if she were fit. What do you think?

Let's talk about movement. Overweight people tend to be more reluctant to physically move. There is a tendency to ask folks to hand you things, to get you things. Over time, what is that going to do to your heart and cardiovascular system? It will become less strong. Your resting heart rate will go up as your cardio condition deteriorates. Your blood pressure will go up. Top athletes have a resting heart rate around 50. Obese folks might be 80 or higher. Athletes have normal to lower than normal blood pressure. Obese folks tend to have high blood pressure. This equals meds and side effects of those meds. Or worse, no meds and arteriosclerosis and death early. As always, **consult your physician before implementing any changes**.

Skin condition. Obese folks can develop diabetes which affects skin health. I've heard of people having amputations due to obesity. Now they don't say, it's because of food addiction, they blame diabetes, which came directly from obesity. You must address this problem. Get help if necessary but get to your correct weight.

The Fit Feeling

Somewhere along the climb back into fitness you will start experiencing a feeling of excitement that you may not have felt in your whole life or perhaps you felt in your past. It is when you start feeling in control of your muscles again, particularly around your abdomen, your core muscles. These have been stretched due to obesity and it is a rush to feel them taut again. I compare it to the feeling of the main character in the movie Predator when he lets out his primal yell to meet the challenge with the predator, with the lit torch in his hand.

It's a somewhat emotional experience to realize that you are about to regain your life at an optimal level of physical condition. In other words, your body fitness at a peak. You are going to love it! It is very exciting, that feeling of strength as you go from being sort of out of shape, not exercising very much, to getting more and more strong. It feels fantastic to be strong again, near your correct weight.

At the same time that you are getting physically stronger, your inner self will get stronger. This "getting fit" is getting in touch with that person, that sense of self, that sense of capability. So feel the excitement of fitness. Envision yourself dressing in your best clothing and new clothing, different clothing that flatters you and accentuates that feeling you have inside of you.

Fading Memories of Obesity

It all seems like so long ago now. I feel so completely different now. I am high energy, look great, feel great and the whole thing of being obese seems like a long time ago. I feel like a fit person and it is a wonderful feeling. I feel so alive and enthusiastic and excited about everything. Anything I want to do, I feel like I can do it. I am bringing energy into every activity, into each interaction with people and it makes for a completely different experience. My new level of fitness is very impactful upon my human relationships and my political capital as well. I am very, very happy that I made the decision to manage my weight. I can't tell you how wonderful it is. It is just night and day. Trust me you will love it.

As I look back at this journey to my right weight, it is hard to believe where I was. I feel great and move well. It is hard to believe there was a time when I could not easily pick up something that I dropped. I had to get down on one knee and then strain to get back to a standing position. I was falling asleep all the time, now I have boundless energy.

It is almost like I felt when I got out of school! Everything is positive. I look different. People treat me differently and I am excited at every interaction with others. There is no more silent indifference. It has been replaced by energetic interaction.

Jump Starting

There are some things that have changed in my lifestyle and habits since I started. These are the new habits that I have established and the DREAM foods that enable me to easily control my caloric balance. Frankly, it no longer takes significant will power to eat correctly. If I had it to do over, I would change to these habits immediately. Remember DREAM foods are Durable, Repeatable, Enjoyable, Affordable and Measurable.

For one, I routinely cook things in advance. I'll cook some chicken or some beef, perhaps some shrimp. I go through the day and when I open the refrigerator there is some meat to snack on or some left over salad. I also sometimes mix the meats with good, slow release vegetables and seasonings.

For example, I have a dish that I frequently make which heavily uses green beans, which are 70 calories per 14 ounce can. That's 5 calories per ounce! Compare that to beef at 40 or chicken at 35. I mix it with some other vegetables like peppers and scallions with some bits of meat. I portion these out in advance and put them in plastic tubs with tops and freeze or refrigerate them for quick, tasty, later heating. I try to go with 200 to 350 calories per tub, or less. The point is to know the count.

I also prepare other DREAM foods such as seasoned chicken pieces of 35 calories each or about 1 ounce.

I have identified some DREAM foods at restaurants and at home. For example:

Tacos – approx. 300 calories

Spicy chicken sandwich (meat only) – approx. 200 calories

Cereal and milk – ½ cup total – approx. 200

2 Tablespoons of ice cream – approx. 150?

Drumstick and chicken thigh — 400 calories fried, 250 baked which I love with garlic salt and pepper.

Steak — 40 calories per ounce (really effective hang time which means durability)

Communicate!

I cannot overstate the importance of other people in this effort. Other people can help or hinder your efforts. Tell them what you are doing. Label your POUNDS foods in the fridge and pantry. Just write "POUNDS!" right on them!

FITME

"FITME" — "Fit (me) Is Truly More Effective"

"FEED" — "Fitness Enhances Effectiveness Dramatically"

As we wrap up, let's do a deeper dive on the impact of fitness on our effectiveness at accomplishing our objectives.

Does being overweight affect our social life? What about our political life, as in our image and reputation? How important is fitness to appearance? Does appearance affect effectiveness? Do you want to be effective? Of course you do!

How important is fitness to intelligence? Alan Turing, the father of the computer, AI and the solver of the Enigma encoding machine which allowed us to win WWII, was an avid runner. He frequently ran tens of miles to work and study. Tesla, the inventor of our modern electric grid, alternating current, ac motors and generators and much more, drew the design for the AC motor on the sand after a long run with a friend. He was an avid long distance runner. Both were very fit, not overweight and both were highly effective. Could it be that their extremely important contributions to mankind had something to do with their fitness?

Optimize your social and political spheres, your health, energy level and mental acuity. Be effective by maintaining your optimal body weight.

Focus on Your Next Meal

As you are on this journey, it can be overwhelming because it is going to take a while. Just as a journey of a thousand miles begins with a single step, so too your journey to reach your correct weight begins with the next thing you put in your mouth. Focus on that next meal. You will make a thousand decisions between now and when you reach your correct weight. Similarly it would take a thousand steps to complete a long walk. Each step takes a decision and the will to take that individual step. Your decision at each meal will take a decision and the will to stay the course during the meal. It does get much easier with time and repetition, just as walking becomes almost effortless over time. Notice how carefully a baby takes those first few steps. So too you must be careful during your meals, especially at the beginning.

Remember, you are losing weight right now if you are not eating or drinking calories! This is because your body is burning calories all the time, continuously. So this is a rate of eating thing. Just don't eat too much at each meal. In fact, under eat. Plan the next meal, nail it down and restate your commitment, "the most important thing I will do today is to manage my caloric intake."

Find your DREAM foods and ease that weight down to your target. Take command of your grocery shopping, watch out for POUNDS situations and especially distracted and social eating! Do it! Enjoy the gift of your life at your best!